I0425004

ISBN: 9781093414530

You can use this book to keep track of your appointment notes. The sections are pretty self-explanatory, and there is no wrong way to use this log.

I've included lots of space to keep notes, but of course feel free to use multiple pages for the same appointment if you need to. You could doodle in the empty space if you don't fill up a page.

BEFORE THE APPOINTMENT   APPOINTMENT DATE: _____

Name of Doctor: _____
Specialty: _____

Primary concern: _____
_____
_____
_____
_____
_____
_____

Related symptoms:_____
_____
_____
_____
_____
_____
_____

Secondary concern:_____
_____
_____
_____
_____
_____
_____

Related symptoms:_____
_____
_____
_____
_____
_____
_____

Follow-up from last appointment:_____
_____
_____
_____
_____
_____
_____

DURING/AFTER APPOINTMENT   DATE: _____

Doctor's advice on primary concern:_____

_____
_____
_____
_____
_____
_____

Doctor's advice on secondary concern:_____

_____
_____
_____
_____
_____
_____

Other notes:

_____
_____
_____
_____
_____
_____
_____
_____
_____
_____
_____
_____
_____
_____
_____
_____
_____
_____
_____
_____
_____
_____
_____
_____

BEFORE THE APPOINTMENT   APPOINTMENT DATE: _____

Name of Doctor: _____
Specialty: _____

Primary concern: _____
_____
_____
_____
_____
_____
_____

Related symptoms: _____
_____
_____
_____
_____
_____
_____
_____

Secondary concern: _____
_____
_____
_____
_____
_____
_____

Related symptoms: _____
_____
_____
_____
_____
_____
_____

Follow-up from last appointment: _____
_____
_____
_____
_____
_____
_____

DURING/AFTER APPOINTMENT   DATE: _____

Doctor's advice on primary concern:_____

_____

_____

_____

_____

_____

_____

Doctor's advice on secondary concern:_____

_____

_____

_____

_____

_____

_____

Other notes:

_____

_____

_____

_____

_____

_____

_____

_____

_____

_____

_____

_____

_____

_____

_____

_____

_____

_____

_____

_____

BEFORE THE APPOINTMENT   APPOINTMENT DATE: _____

Name of Doctor: _____

Specialty: _____

Primary concern: _____

_____

_____

_____

_____

_____

_____

Related symptoms: _____

_____

_____

_____

_____

_____

_____

Secondary concern: _____

_____

_____

_____

_____

_____

_____

Related symptoms: _____

_____

_____

_____

_____

_____

_____

Follow-up from last appointment: _____

_____

_____

_____

_____

_____

_____

DURING/AFTER APPOINTMENT   DATE: _____

Doctor's advice on primary concern:_____

_____
_____
_____
_____
_____
_____
_____

Doctor's advice on secondary concern:_____

_____
_____
_____
_____
_____
_____
_____

Other notes:

_____
_____
_____
_____
_____
_____
_____
_____
_____
_____
_____
_____
_____
_____
_____
_____
_____
_____
_____
_____
_____
_____
_____

BEFORE THE APPOINTMENT   APPOINTMENT DATE: _____

Name of Doctor: _____

Specialty: _____

Primary concern: _____

_____
_____
_____
_____
_____
_____

Related symptoms:_____

_____
_____
_____
_____
_____
_____

Secondary concern:_____

_____
_____
_____
_____
_____
_____

Related symptoms:_____

_____
_____
_____
_____
_____
_____

Follow-up from last appointment:_____

_____
_____
_____
_____
_____
_____

DURING/AFTER APPOINTMENT

DATE: _____

Doctor's advice on primary concern:_____

_____

_____

_____

_____

_____

_____

Doctor's advice on secondary concern:_____

_____

_____

_____

_____

_____

_____

Other notes:

_____

_____

_____

_____

_____

_____

_____

_____

_____

_____

_____

_____

_____

_____

_____

_____

_____

_____

_____

_____

_____

_____

_____

BEFORE THE APPOINTMENT   APPOINTMENT DATE: _____

Name of Doctor: _____

Specialty: _____

Primary concern: _____

_____
_____
_____
_____
_____
_____

Related symptoms:_____

_____
_____
_____
_____
_____
_____

Secondary concern:_____

_____
_____
_____
_____
_____
_____

Related symptoms:_____

_____
_____
_____
_____
_____
_____

Follow-up from last appointment:_____

_____
_____
_____
_____
_____
_____

DURING/AFTER APPOINTMENT

DATE: _____

Doctor's advice on primary concern:_____

_____
_____
_____
_____
_____
_____

Doctor's advice on secondary concern:_____

_____
_____
_____
_____
_____
_____

Other notes:

_____
_____
_____
_____
_____
_____
_____
_____
_____
_____
_____
_____
_____
_____
_____
_____
_____
_____
_____
_____
_____
_____
_____

BEFORE THE APPOINTMENT   APPOINTMENT DATE: _____

Name of Doctor: _____

Specialty: _____

Primary concern: _____
_____
_____
_____
_____
_____
_____

Related symptoms:_____
_____
_____
_____
_____
_____
_____

Secondary concern:_____
_____
_____
_____
_____
_____
_____

Related symptoms:_____
_____
_____
_____
_____
_____
_____

Follow-up from last appointment:_____
_____
_____
_____
_____
_____
_____

DURING/AFTER APPOINTMENT   DATE: _____

Doctor's advice on primary concern:_____

_____
_____
_____
_____
_____
_____

Doctor's advice on secondary concern:_____

_____
_____
_____
_____
_____
_____

Other notes:

_____
_____
_____
_____
_____
_____
_____
_____
_____
_____
_____
_____
_____
_____
_____
_____
_____
_____
_____
_____
_____
_____
_____
_____

BEFORE THE APPOINTMENT   APPOINTMENT DATE: _____

Name of Doctor: _____

Specialty: _____

Primary concern: _____

_____
_____
_____
_____
_____
_____

Related symptoms: _____

_____
_____
_____
_____
_____
_____

Secondary concern: _____

_____
_____
_____
_____
_____

Related symptoms: _____

_____
_____
_____
_____
_____

Follow-up from last appointment: _____

_____
_____
_____
_____
_____

DURING/AFTER APPOINTMENT   DATE: _____

Doctor's advice on primary concern:_____

_____
_____
_____
_____
_____
_____
_____

Doctor's advice on secondary concern:_____

_____
_____
_____
_____
_____
_____

Other notes:

_____
_____
_____
_____
_____
_____
_____
_____
_____
_____
_____
_____
_____
_____
_____
_____
_____
_____
_____
_____
_____

BEFORE THE APPOINTMENT   APPOINTMENT DATE: _____

Name of Doctor: _____
Specialty: _____

Primary concern: _____
_____
_____
_____
_____
_____
_____

Related symptoms:_____
_____
_____
_____
_____
_____
_____

Secondary concern:_____
_____
_____
_____
_____
_____
_____

Related symptoms:_____
_____
_____
_____
_____
_____
_____

Follow-up from last appointment:_____
_____
_____
_____
_____
_____
_____

DURING/AFTER APPOINTMENT   DATE: _____

Doctor's advice on primary concern:_____

_____
_____
_____
_____
_____
_____

Doctor's advice on secondary concern:_____

_____
_____
_____
_____
_____
_____

Other notes:

_____
_____
_____
_____
_____
_____
_____
_____
_____
_____
_____
_____
_____
_____
_____
_____
_____
_____
_____
_____
_____
_____
_____

BEFORE THE APPOINTMENT   APPOINTMENT DATE: _____

Name of Doctor: _____
Specialty: _____

Primary concern: _____
_____
_____
_____
_____
_____
_____

Related symptoms: _____
_____
_____
_____
_____
_____
_____

Secondary concern: _____
_____
_____
_____
_____
_____
_____

Related symptoms: _____
_____
_____
_____
_____
_____
_____

Follow-up from last appointment: _____
_____
_____
_____
_____
_____
_____

DURING/AFTER APPOINTMENT   DATE: _____

Doctor's advice on primary concern: _____
_____
_____
_____
_____
_____
_____

Doctor's advice on secondary concern: _____
_____
_____
_____
_____
_____
_____

Other notes:
_____
_____
_____
_____
_____
_____
_____
_____
_____
_____
_____
_____
_____
_____
_____
_____
_____
_____
_____
_____
_____
_____

BEFORE THE APPOINTMENT   APPOINTMENT DATE: _____

Name of Doctor: _____

Specialty: _____

    Primary concern: _____

_____

_____

_____

_____

_____

_____

    Related symptoms:_____

_____

_____

_____

_____

_____

_____

    Secondary concern:_____

_____

_____

_____

_____

_____

_____

    Related symptoms:_____

_____

_____

_____

_____

_____

_____

    Follow-up from last appointment:_____

_____

_____

_____

_____

_____

_____

DURING/AFTER APPOINTMENT

DATE: _____

Doctor's advice on primary concern:_____

_____
_____
_____
_____
_____
_____

Doctor's advice on secondary concern:_____

_____
_____
_____
_____
_____
_____

Other notes:

_____
_____
_____
_____
_____
_____
_____
_____
_____
_____
_____
_____
_____
_____
_____
_____
_____
_____
_____
_____
_____
_____
_____
_____
_____

BEFORE THE APPOINTMENT   APPOINTMENT DATE: _____

Name of Doctor: _____
Specialty: _____

Primary concern: _____
_____
_____
_____
_____
_____
_____

Related symptoms: _____
_____
_____
_____
_____
_____
_____

Secondary concern: _____
_____
_____
_____
_____
_____
_____

Related symptoms: _____
_____
_____
_____
_____
_____
_____

Follow-up from last appointment: _____
_____
_____
_____
_____
_____
_____

DURING/AFTER APPOINTMENT   DATE: _____

Doctor's advice on primary concern:_____

_____
_____
_____
_____
_____
_____

Doctor's advice on secondary concern:_____

_____
_____
_____
_____
_____
_____

Other notes:

_____
_____
_____
_____
_____
_____
_____
_____
_____
_____
_____
_____
_____
_____
_____
_____
_____
_____
_____
_____
_____
_____
_____

BEFORE THE APPOINTMENT   APPOINTMENT DATE: _____

Name of Doctor: _____

Specialty: _____

Primary concern: _____

_____
_____
_____
_____
_____
_____

Related symptoms:_____

_____
_____
_____
_____
_____
_____

Secondary concern:_____

_____
_____
_____
_____
_____

Related symptoms:_____

_____
_____
_____
_____
_____

Follow-up from last appointment:_____

_____
_____
_____
_____
_____

DURING/AFTER APPOINTMENT   DATE: _____

Doctor's advice on primary concern:_____
_____
_____
_____
_____
_____
_____

Doctor's advice on secondary concern:_____
_____
_____
_____
_____
_____
_____

Other notes:
_____
_____
_____
_____
_____
_____
_____
_____
_____
_____
_____
_____
_____
_____
_____
_____
_____
_____
_____
_____
_____

BEFORE THE APPOINTMENT   APPOINTMENT DATE: _____

Name of Doctor: _____

Specialty: _____

Primary concern: _____

_____
_____
_____
_____
_____
_____

Related symptoms: _____

_____
_____
_____
_____
_____
_____

Secondary concern: _____

_____
_____
_____
_____
_____
_____

Related symptoms: _____

_____
_____
_____
_____
_____
_____

Follow-up from last appointment: _____

_____
_____
_____
_____
_____
_____

DURING/AFTER APPOINTMENT   DATE: _____

Doctor's advice on primary concern:_____

_____
_____
_____
_____
_____
_____
_____

Doctor's advice on secondary concern:_____

_____
_____
_____
_____
_____
_____
_____

Other notes:

_____
_____
_____
_____
_____
_____
_____
_____
_____
_____
_____
_____
_____
_____
_____
_____
_____
_____
_____
_____
_____
_____
_____
_____

BEFORE THE APPOINTMENT   APPOINTMENT DATE: _____

Name of Doctor: _____
Specialty: _____

Primary concern: _____
_____
_____
_____
_____
_____
_____

Related symptoms:_____
_____
_____
_____
_____
_____
_____

Secondary concern:_____
_____
_____
_____
_____
_____
_____

Related symptoms:_____
_____
_____
_____
_____
_____
_____

Follow-up from last appointment:_____
_____
_____
_____
_____
_____
_____

DURING/AFTER APPOINTMENT   DATE: _____

Doctor's advice on primary concern:_____

_____
_____
_____
_____
_____
_____

Doctor's advice on secondary concern:_____

_____
_____
_____
_____
_____
_____

Other notes:

_____
_____
_____
_____
_____
_____
_____
_____
_____
_____
_____
_____
_____
_____
_____
_____
_____
_____
_____
_____
_____
_____
_____
_____

BEFORE THE APPOINTMENT   APPOINTMENT DATE: _____

Name of Doctor: _____

Specialty: _____

Primary concern: _____

_____
_____
_____
_____
_____
_____

Related symptoms: _____

_____
_____
_____
_____
_____
_____

Secondary concern: _____

_____
_____
_____
_____
_____
_____

Related symptoms: _____

_____
_____
_____
_____
_____

Follow-up from last appointment: _____

_____
_____
_____
_____
_____

DURING/AFTER APPOINTMENT   DATE: _____

Doctor's advice on primary concern:_____

_____
_____
_____
_____
_____
_____

Doctor's advice on secondary concern:_____

_____
_____
_____
_____
_____
_____

Other notes:

_____
_____
_____
_____
_____
_____
_____
_____
_____
_____
_____
_____
_____
_____
_____
_____
_____
_____
_____
_____
_____
_____

BEFORE THE APPOINTMENT   APPOINTMENT DATE: _____

Name of Doctor: _____

Specialty: _____

Primary concern: _____

_____
_____
_____
_____
_____
_____

Related symptoms: _____

_____
_____
_____
_____
_____
_____

Secondary concern: _____

_____
_____
_____
_____
_____
_____

Related symptoms: _____

_____
_____
_____
_____
_____
_____

Follow-up from last appointment: _____

_____
_____
_____
_____
_____
_____

DURING/AFTER APPOINTMENT   DATE: _____

Doctor's advice on primary concern:_____

_____

_____

_____

_____

_____

_____

Doctor's advice on secondary concern:_____

_____

_____

_____

_____

_____

_____

Other notes:

_____

_____

_____

_____

_____

_____

_____

_____

_____

_____

_____

_____

_____

_____

_____

_____

_____

_____

_____

_____

_____

BEFORE THE APPOINTMENT   APPOINTMENT DATE: _____

Name of Doctor: _____
Specialty: _____

Primary concern: _____
_____
_____
_____
_____
_____
_____

Related symptoms:_____
_____
_____
_____
_____
_____
_____

Secondary concern:_____
_____
_____
_____
_____
_____
_____

Related symptoms:_____
_____
_____
_____
_____
_____
_____

Follow-up from last appointment:_____
_____
_____
_____
_____
_____

DURING/AFTER APPOINTMENT

DATE: _____

Doctor's advice on primary concern:_____

_____
_____
_____
_____
_____
_____

Doctor's advice on secondary concern:_____

_____
_____
_____
_____
_____
_____

Other notes:

_____
_____
_____
_____
_____
_____
_____
_____
_____
_____
_____
_____
_____
_____
_____
_____
_____
_____
_____
_____
_____
_____
_____

BEFORE THE APPOINTMENT   APPOINTMENT DATE: _____

Name of Doctor: _____

Specialty: _____

   Primary concern: _____

_____
_____
_____
_____
_____
_____

   Related symptoms: _____

_____
_____
_____
_____
_____
_____

   Secondary concern: _____

_____
_____
_____
_____
_____

   Related symptoms: _____

_____
_____
_____
_____
_____
_____

   Follow-up from last appointment: _____

_____
_____
_____
_____
_____

DURING/AFTER APPOINTMENT   DATE: _____

Doctor's advice on primary concern:_____

_____
_____
_____
_____
_____
_____

Doctor's advice on secondary concern:_____

_____
_____
_____
_____
_____
_____

Other notes:

_____
_____
_____
_____
_____
_____
_____
_____
_____
_____
_____
_____
_____
_____
_____
_____
_____
_____
_____
_____
_____
_____
_____
_____

BEFORE THE APPOINTMENT   APPOINTMENT DATE: _____

Name of Doctor: _____

Specialty: _____

Primary concern: _____

_____
_____
_____
_____
_____
_____

Related symptoms:_____

_____
_____
_____
_____
_____
_____

Secondary concern:_____

_____
_____
_____
_____
_____

Related symptoms:_____

_____
_____
_____
_____
_____
_____

Follow-up from last appointment:_____

_____
_____
_____
_____
_____

DURING/AFTER APPOINTMENT   DATE: _____

Doctor's advice on primary concern:_____

_____
_____
_____
_____
_____
_____
_____

Doctor's advice on secondary concern:_____

_____
_____
_____
_____
_____
_____

Other notes:

_____
_____
_____
_____
_____
_____
_____
_____
_____
_____
_____
_____
_____
_____
_____
_____
_____
_____
_____
_____
_____
_____
_____

BEFORE THE APPOINTMENT   APPOINTMENT DATE: _____

Name of Doctor: _____

Specialty: _____

Primary concern: _____

_____
_____
_____
_____
_____
_____

Related symptoms:_____

_____
_____
_____
_____
_____
_____

Secondary concern:_____

_____
_____
_____
_____
_____
_____

Related symptoms:_____

_____
_____
_____
_____
_____
_____

Follow-up from last appointment:_____

_____
_____
_____
_____
_____
_____

DURING/AFTER APPOINTMENT   DATE: _____

Doctor's advice on primary concern:_____
_____
_____
_____
_____
_____
_____

Doctor's advice on secondary concern:_____
_____
_____
_____
_____
_____
_____

Other notes:
_____
_____
_____
_____
_____
_____
_____
_____
_____
_____
_____
_____
_____
_____
_____
_____
_____
_____
_____
_____
_____
_____

BEFORE THE APPOINTMENT   APPOINTMENT DATE: _____

Name of Doctor: _____

Specialty: _____

Primary concern: _____

_____
_____
_____
_____
_____
_____

Related symptoms: _____

_____
_____
_____
_____
_____
_____

Secondary concern: _____

_____
_____
_____
_____
_____

Related symptoms: _____

_____
_____
_____
_____
_____

Follow-up from last appointment: _____

_____
_____
_____
_____
_____

DURING/AFTER APPOINTMENT   DATE: _____

Doctor's advice on primary concern:_____
_____
_____
_____
_____
_____
_____

Doctor's advice on secondary concern:_____
_____
_____
_____
_____
_____

Other notes:
_____
_____
_____
_____
_____
_____
_____
_____
_____
_____
_____
_____
_____
_____
_____
_____
_____
_____
_____
_____

BEFORE THE APPOINTMENT   APPOINTMENT DATE: _____

Name of Doctor: _____

Specialty: _____

Primary concern: _____
_____
_____
_____
_____
_____
_____

Related symptoms: _____
_____
_____
_____
_____
_____
_____

Secondary concern: _____
_____
_____
_____
_____
_____

Related symptoms: _____
_____
_____
_____
_____
_____

Follow-up from last appointment: _____
_____
_____
_____
_____
_____

DURING/AFTER APPOINTMENT   DATE: _____

Doctor's advice on primary concern:_____

_____
_____
_____
_____
_____
_____

Doctor's advice on secondary concern:_____

_____
_____
_____
_____
_____
_____

Other notes:

_____
_____
_____
_____
_____
_____
_____
_____
_____
_____
_____
_____
_____
_____
_____
_____
_____
_____
_____
_____
_____
_____

BEFORE THE APPOINTMENT   APPOINTMENT DATE: _____

Name of Doctor: _____
Specialty: _____

Primary concern: _____
_____
_____
_____
_____
_____
_____

Related symptoms:_____
_____
_____
_____
_____
_____
_____

Secondary concern:_____
_____
_____
_____
_____
_____

Related symptoms:_____
_____
_____
_____
_____
_____

Follow-up from last appointment:_____
_____
_____
_____
_____
_____

DURING/AFTER APPOINTMENT   DATE: _____

Doctor's advice on primary concern:_____
_____
_____
_____
_____
_____
_____

Doctor's advice on secondary concern:_____
_____
_____
_____
_____
_____
_____

Other notes:
_____
_____
_____
_____
_____
_____
_____
_____
_____
_____
_____
_____
_____
_____
_____
_____
_____
_____
_____
_____
_____
_____
_____

BEFORE THE APPOINTMENT   APPOINTMENT DATE: _____

Name of Doctor: _____
Specialty: _____

Primary concern: _____
_____
_____
_____
_____
_____
_____

Related symptoms:_____
_____
_____
_____
_____
_____
_____

Secondary concern:_____
_____
_____
_____
_____
_____

Related symptoms:_____
_____
_____
_____
_____
_____
_____

Follow-up from last appointment:_____
_____
_____
_____
_____
_____

DURING/AFTER APPOINTMENT   DATE: _____

Doctor's advice on primary concern:_____
_____
_____
_____
_____
_____
_____

Doctor's advice on secondary concern:_____
_____
_____
_____
_____
_____
_____

Other notes:
_____
_____
_____
_____
_____
_____
_____
_____
_____
_____
_____
_____
_____
_____
_____
_____
_____
_____
_____
_____
_____
_____

BEFORE THE APPOINTMENT   APPOINTMENT DATE: _____

Name of Doctor: _____
Specialty: _____

Primary concern: _____
_____
_____
_____
_____
_____
_____
_____

Related symptoms:_____
_____
_____
_____
_____
_____
_____
_____

Secondary concern:_____
_____
_____
_____
_____
_____
_____

Related symptoms:_____
_____
_____
_____
_____
_____
_____

Follow-up from last appointment:_____
_____
_____
_____
_____
_____
_____

DURING/AFTER APPOINTMENT   DATE: _____

Doctor's advice on primary concern:_____

_____
_____
_____
_____
_____
_____
_____

Doctor's advice on secondary concern:_____

_____
_____
_____
_____
_____
_____
_____

Other notes:

_____
_____
_____
_____
_____
_____
_____
_____
_____
_____
_____
_____
_____
_____
_____
_____
_____
_____
_____
_____
_____
_____
_____
_____
_____

BEFORE THE APPOINTMENT   APPOINTMENT DATE: _____

Name of Doctor: _____

Specialty: _____

Primary concern: _____
_____
_____
_____
_____
_____
_____

Related symptoms: _____
_____
_____
_____
_____
_____
_____

Secondary concern: _____
_____
_____
_____
_____
_____
_____

Related symptoms: _____
_____
_____
_____
_____
_____
_____

Follow-up from last appointment: _____
_____
_____
_____
_____
_____

DURING/AFTER APPOINTMENT   DATE: _____

Doctor's advice on primary concern:_____

_____

_____

_____

_____

_____

_____

Doctor's advice on secondary concern:_____

_____

_____

_____

_____

_____

_____

Other notes:

_____

_____

_____

_____

_____

_____

_____

_____

_____

_____

_____

_____

_____

_____

_____

_____

_____

_____

_____

_____

_____

_____

_____

_____

BEFORE THE APPOINTMENT   APPOINTMENT DATE: _____

Name of Doctor: _____
Specialty: _____

Primary concern: _____
_____
_____
_____
_____
_____
_____

Related symptoms: _____
_____
_____
_____
_____
_____
_____

Secondary concern: _____
_____
_____
_____
_____
_____
_____

Related symptoms: _____
_____
_____
_____
_____
_____
_____

Follow-up from last appointment: _____
_____
_____
_____
_____
_____
_____

DURING/AFTER APPOINTMENT   DATE: _____

Doctor's advice on primary concern:_____

_____

_____

_____

_____

_____

_____

Doctor's advice on secondary concern:_____

_____

_____

_____

_____

_____

_____

Other notes:

_____

_____

_____

_____

_____

_____

_____

_____

_____

_____

_____

_____

_____

_____

_____

_____

_____

_____

_____

_____

_____

_____

BEFORE THE APPOINTMENT   APPOINTMENT DATE: _____

Name of Doctor: _____

Specialty: _____

Primary concern: _____

_____
_____
_____
_____
_____
_____

Related symptoms:_____

_____
_____
_____
_____
_____
_____

Secondary concern:_____

_____
_____
_____
_____
_____
_____

Related symptoms:_____

_____
_____
_____
_____
_____
_____

Follow-up from last appointment:_____

_____
_____
_____
_____
_____
_____

DURING/AFTER APPOINTMENT   DATE: _____

Doctor's advice on primary concern:_____
_____
_____
_____
_____
_____
_____

Doctor's advice on secondary concern:_____
_____
_____
_____
_____
_____
_____

Other notes:
_____
_____
_____
_____
_____
_____
_____
_____
_____
_____
_____
_____
_____
_____
_____
_____
_____
_____
_____
_____

BEFORE THE APPOINTMENT   APPOINTMENT DATE: _____

Name of Doctor: _____
Specialty: _____

Primary concern: _____
_____
_____
_____
_____
_____
_____

Related symptoms:_____
_____
_____
_____
_____
_____
_____

Secondary concern:_____
_____
_____
_____
_____
_____
_____

Related symptoms:_____
_____
_____
_____
_____
_____

Follow-up from last appointment:_____
_____
_____
_____
_____
_____

DURING/AFTER APPOINTMENT

DATE: _____

Doctor's advice on primary concern:_____

_____
_____
_____
_____
_____
_____

Doctor's advice on secondary concern:_____

_____
_____
_____
_____
_____
_____

Other notes:

_____
_____
_____
_____
_____
_____
_____
_____
_____
_____
_____
_____
_____
_____
_____
_____
_____
_____
_____
_____
_____
_____
_____
_____

BEFORE THE APPOINTMENT   APPOINTMENT DATE: _____

Name of Doctor: _____
Specialty: _____

Primary concern: _____
_____
_____
_____
_____
_____
_____

Related symptoms: _____
_____
_____
_____
_____
_____
_____

Secondary concern: _____
_____
_____
_____
_____
_____
_____

Related symptoms: _____
_____
_____
_____
_____
_____
_____

Follow-up from last appointment: _____
_____
_____
_____
_____
_____
_____

DURING/AFTER APPOINTMENT   DATE: _____

Doctor's advice on primary concern:_____

_____
_____
_____
_____
_____
_____

Doctor's advice on secondary concern:_____

_____
_____
_____
_____
_____
_____

Other notes:

_____
_____
_____
_____
_____
_____
_____
_____
_____
_____
_____
_____
_____
_____
_____
_____
_____
_____
_____
_____
_____
_____
_____

BEFORE THE APPOINTMENT   APPOINTMENT DATE: _____

Name of Doctor: _____

Specialty: _____

Primary concern: _____

_____
_____
_____
_____
_____
_____

Related symptoms: _____

_____
_____
_____
_____
_____
_____

Secondary concern: _____

_____
_____
_____
_____
_____

Related symptoms: _____

_____
_____
_____
_____
_____
_____

Follow-up from last appointment: _____

_____
_____
_____
_____
_____

DURING/AFTER APPOINTMENT   DATE: _____

Doctor's advice on primary concern:_____
_____
_____
_____
_____
_____
_____

Doctor's advice on secondary concern:_____
_____
_____
_____
_____
_____
_____

Other notes:
_____
_____
_____
_____
_____
_____
_____
_____
_____
_____
_____
_____
_____
_____
_____
_____
_____
_____
_____
_____
_____
_____
_____
_____

BEFORE THE APPOINTMENT   APPOINTMENT DATE: _____

Name of Doctor: _____

Specialty: _____

Primary concern: _____
_____
_____
_____
_____
_____
_____

Related symptoms: _____
_____
_____
_____
_____
_____
_____

Secondary concern: _____
_____
_____
_____
_____
_____
_____

Related symptoms: _____
_____
_____
_____
_____
_____
_____

Follow-up from last appointment: _____
_____
_____
_____
_____
_____
_____

DURING/AFTER APPOINTMENT

DATE: _____

Doctor's advice on primary concern: _____

_____
_____
_____
_____
_____
_____

Doctor's advice on secondary concern: _____

_____
_____
_____
_____
_____
_____

Other notes:

_____
_____
_____
_____
_____
_____
_____
_____
_____
_____
_____
_____
_____
_____
_____
_____
_____
_____
_____
_____
_____
_____
_____

BEFORE THE APPOINTMENT   APPOINTMENT DATE: _____

Name of Doctor: _____

Specialty: _____

Primary concern: _____

_____
_____
_____
_____
_____
_____

Related symptoms: _____

_____
_____
_____
_____
_____
_____

Secondary concern: _____

_____
_____
_____
_____
_____
_____

Related symptoms: _____

_____
_____
_____
_____
_____
_____

Follow-up from last appointment: _____

_____
_____
_____
_____
_____

DURING/AFTER APPOINTMENT   DATE: _____

Doctor's advice on primary concern:_____

_____

_____

_____

_____

_____

_____

Doctor's advice on secondary concern:_____

_____

_____

_____

_____

_____

_____

Other notes:

_____

_____

_____

_____

_____

_____

_____

_____

_____

_____

_____

_____

_____

_____

_____

_____

_____

_____

_____

_____

BEFORE THE APPOINTMENT   APPOINTMENT DATE: _____

Name of Doctor: _____
Specialty: _____

Primary concern: _____
_____
_____
_____
_____
_____
_____

Related symptoms: _____
_____
_____
_____
_____
_____
_____

Secondary concern: _____
_____
_____
_____
_____
_____
_____

Related symptoms: _____
_____
_____
_____
_____
_____

Follow-up from last appointment: _____
_____
_____
_____
_____
_____
_____

DURING/AFTER APPOINTMENT   DATE: _____

Doctor's advice on primary concern:_____
_____
_____
_____
_____
_____
_____

Doctor's advice on secondary concern:_____
_____
_____
_____
_____
_____
_____

Other notes:
_____
_____
_____
_____
_____
_____
_____
_____
_____
_____
_____
_____
_____
_____
_____
_____
_____
_____
_____
_____
_____
_____

BEFORE THE APPOINTMENT   APPOINTMENT DATE: _____

Name of Doctor: _____

Specialty: _____

Primary concern: _____
_____
_____
_____
_____
_____
_____

Related symptoms: _____
_____
_____
_____
_____
_____
_____

Secondary concern: _____
_____
_____
_____
_____
_____
_____

Related symptoms: _____
_____
_____
_____
_____
_____
_____

Follow-up from last appointment: _____
_____
_____
_____
_____
_____
_____

DURING/AFTER APPOINTMENT   DATE: _____

Doctor's advice on primary concern:_____

_____
_____
_____
_____
_____
_____

Doctor's advice on secondary concern:_____

_____
_____
_____
_____
_____
_____

Other notes:

_____
_____
_____
_____
_____
_____
_____
_____
_____
_____
_____
_____
_____
_____
_____
_____
_____
_____
_____
_____
_____
_____
_____

BEFORE THE APPOINTMENT   APPOINTMENT DATE: _____

Name of Doctor: _____
Specialty: _____

Primary concern: _____
_____
_____
_____
_____
_____
_____

Related symptoms: _____
_____
_____
_____
_____
_____
_____

Secondary concern: _____
_____
_____
_____
_____
_____
_____

Related symptoms: _____
_____
_____
_____
_____
_____
_____

Follow-up from last appointment: _____
_____
_____
_____
_____
_____
_____

DURING/AFTER APPOINTMENT   DATE: _____

Doctor's advice on primary concern:_____

_____
_____
_____
_____
_____
_____

Doctor's advice on secondary concern:_____

_____
_____
_____
_____
_____
_____

Other notes:

_____
_____
_____
_____
_____
_____
_____
_____
_____
_____
_____
_____
_____
_____
_____
_____
_____
_____
_____
_____
_____
_____
_____
_____
_____

BEFORE THE APPOINTMENT   APPOINTMENT DATE: _____

Name of Doctor: _____

Specialty: _____

Primary concern: _____
_____
_____
_____
_____
_____
_____

Related symptoms:_____
_____
_____
_____
_____
_____
_____

Secondary concern:_____
_____
_____
_____
_____
_____
_____

Related symptoms:_____
_____
_____
_____
_____
_____
_____

Follow-up from last appointment:_____
_____
_____
_____
_____
_____
_____

DURING/AFTER APPOINTMENT

DATE: _____

Doctor's advice on primary concern:_____

_____
_____
_____
_____
_____
_____

Doctor's advice on secondary concern:_____

_____
_____
_____
_____
_____
_____

Other notes:

_____
_____
_____
_____
_____
_____
_____
_____
_____
_____
_____
_____
_____
_____
_____
_____
_____
_____
_____
_____
_____
_____

BEFORE THE APPOINTMENT   APPOINTMENT DATE: _____

Name of Doctor: _____

Specialty: _____

Primary concern: _____
_____
_____
_____
_____
_____
_____

Related symptoms:_____
_____
_____
_____
_____
_____
_____

Secondary concern:_____
_____
_____
_____
_____
_____
_____

Related symptoms:_____
_____
_____
_____
_____
_____
_____

Follow-up from last appointment:_____
_____
_____
_____
_____
_____
_____

DURING/AFTER APPOINTMENT

DATE: _____

Doctor's advice on primary concern:_____

_____
_____
_____
_____
_____
_____

Doctor's advice on secondary concern:_____

_____
_____
_____
_____
_____
_____

Other notes:

_____
_____
_____
_____
_____
_____
_____
_____
_____
_____
_____
_____
_____
_____
_____
_____
_____
_____
_____
_____
_____
_____

BEFORE THE APPOINTMENT   APPOINTMENT DATE: _____

Name of Doctor: _____
Specialty: _____

Primary concern: _____
_____
_____
_____
_____
_____
_____

Related symptoms: _____
_____
_____
_____
_____
_____
_____
_____

Secondary concern: _____
_____
_____
_____
_____
_____
_____

Related symptoms: _____
_____
_____
_____
_____
_____
_____

Follow-up from last appointment: _____
_____
_____
_____
_____
_____
_____

DURING/AFTER APPOINTMENT   DATE: _____

Doctor's advice on primary concern:_____

_____
_____
_____
_____
_____
_____

Doctor's advice on secondary concern:_____

_____
_____
_____
_____
_____
_____

Other notes:

_____
_____
_____
_____
_____
_____
_____
_____
_____
_____
_____
_____
_____
_____
_____
_____
_____
_____
_____
_____
_____
_____

BEFORE THE APPOINTMENT   APPOINTMENT DATE: _____

Name of Doctor: _____

Specialty: _____

Primary concern: _____
_____
_____
_____
_____
_____
_____

Related symptoms: _____
_____
_____
_____
_____
_____
_____

Secondary concern: _____
_____
_____
_____
_____
_____

Related symptoms: _____
_____
_____
_____
_____
_____
_____

Follow-up from last appointment: _____
_____
_____
_____
_____
_____
_____

DURING/AFTER APPOINTMENT   DATE: _____

Doctor's advice on primary concern:_____

_____

_____

_____

_____

_____

_____

Doctor's advice on secondary concern:_____

_____

_____

_____

_____

_____

_____

Other notes:

_____

_____

_____

_____

_____

_____

_____

_____

_____

_____

_____

_____

_____

_____

_____

_____

_____

_____

_____

_____

_____

_____

BEFORE THE APPOINTMENT   APPOINTMENT DATE: _____

Name of Doctor: _____

Specialty: _____

Primary concern: _____

_____
_____
_____
_____
_____
_____

Related symptoms: _____

_____
_____
_____
_____
_____
_____

Secondary concern: _____

_____
_____
_____
_____
_____
_____

Related symptoms: _____

_____
_____
_____
_____
_____
_____

Follow-up from last appointment: _____

_____
_____
_____
_____
_____
_____

DURING/AFTER APPOINTMENT   DATE: _____

Doctor's advice on primary concern:_____
_____
_____
_____
_____
_____
_____

Doctor's advice on secondary concern:_____
_____
_____
_____
_____
_____
_____

Other notes:
_____
_____
_____
_____
_____
_____
_____
_____
_____
_____
_____
_____
_____
_____
_____
_____
_____
_____
_____
_____

BEFORE THE APPOINTMENT   APPOINTMENT DATE: _____

Name of Doctor: _____
Specialty: _____

Primary concern: _____
_____
_____
_____
_____
_____
_____

Related symptoms: _____
_____
_____
_____
_____
_____
_____

Secondary concern: _____
_____
_____
_____
_____
_____

Related symptoms: _____
_____
_____
_____
_____
_____

Follow-up from last appointment: _____
_____
_____
_____
_____
_____

DURING/AFTER APPOINTMENT   DATE: _____

Doctor's advice on primary concern:_____
_____
_____
_____
_____
_____
_____

Doctor's advice on secondary concern:_____
_____
_____
_____
_____
_____
_____

Other notes:
_____
_____
_____
_____
_____
_____
_____
_____
_____
_____
_____
_____
_____
_____
_____
_____
_____
_____
_____
_____
_____
_____
_____

BEFORE THE APPOINTMENT   APPOINTMENT DATE: _____

Name of Doctor: _____
Specialty: _____

Primary concern: _____
_____
_____
_____
_____
_____
_____

Related symptoms:_____
_____
_____
_____
_____
_____
_____

Secondary concern:_____
_____
_____
_____
_____
_____
_____

Related symptoms:_____
_____
_____
_____
_____
_____
_____

Follow-up from last appointment:_____
_____
_____
_____
_____
_____
_____

DURING/AFTER APPOINTMENT

DATE: _____

Doctor's advice on primary concern:_____

_____
_____
_____
_____
_____
_____

Doctor's advice on secondary concern:_____

_____
_____
_____
_____
_____
_____

Other notes:

_____
_____
_____
_____
_____
_____
_____
_____
_____
_____
_____
_____
_____
_____
_____
_____
_____
_____
_____
_____
_____

BEFORE THE APPOINTMENT   APPOINTMENT DATE: _____

Name of Doctor: _____

Specialty: _____

Primary concern: _____

_____
_____
_____
_____
_____
_____

Related symptoms:_____

_____
_____
_____
_____
_____
_____

Secondary concern:_____

_____
_____
_____
_____
_____
_____

Related symptoms:_____

_____
_____
_____
_____
_____
_____

Follow-up from last appointment:_____

_____
_____
_____
_____
_____

DURING/AFTER APPOINTMENT   DATE: _____

Doctor's advice on primary concern:_____
_____
_____
_____
_____
_____
_____

Doctor's advice on secondary concern:_____
_____
_____
_____
_____
_____
_____

Other notes:
_____
_____
_____
_____
_____
_____
_____
_____
_____
_____
_____
_____
_____
_____
_____
_____
_____
_____
_____
_____
_____
_____
_____

BEFORE THE APPOINTMENT   APPOINTMENT DATE: _____

Name of Doctor: _____

Specialty: _____

Primary concern: _____

_____
_____
_____
_____
_____
_____

Related symptoms: _____

_____
_____
_____
_____
_____
_____

Secondary concern: _____

_____
_____
_____
_____
_____

Related symptoms: _____

_____
_____
_____
_____
_____

Follow-up from last appointment: _____

_____
_____
_____
_____
_____

DURING/AFTER APPOINTMENT   DATE: _____

Doctor's advice on primary concern:_____

_____
_____
_____
_____
_____
_____

Doctor's advice on secondary concern:_____

_____
_____
_____
_____
_____
_____

Other notes:

_____
_____
_____
_____
_____
_____
_____
_____
_____
_____
_____
_____
_____
_____
_____
_____
_____
_____
_____
_____
_____
_____
_____
_____

BEFORE THE APPOINTMENT   APPOINTMENT DATE: _____

Name of Doctor: _____

Specialty: _____

Primary concern: _____
_____
_____
_____
_____
_____
_____

Related symptoms: _____
_____
_____
_____
_____
_____
_____

Secondary concern: _____
_____
_____
_____
_____
_____
_____

Related symptoms: _____
_____
_____
_____
_____
_____
_____

Follow-up from last appointment: _____
_____
_____
_____
_____
_____
_____

DURING/AFTER APPOINTMENT

DATE: _____

Doctor's advice on primary concern:_____

_____
_____
_____
_____
_____
_____

Doctor's advice on secondary concern:_____

_____
_____
_____
_____
_____
_____

Other notes:

_____
_____
_____
_____
_____
_____
_____
_____
_____
_____
_____
_____
_____
_____
_____
_____
_____
_____
_____
_____
_____
_____

BEFORE THE APPOINTMENT   APPOINTMENT DATE: _____

Name of Doctor: _____

Specialty: _____

Primary concern: _____

_____
_____
_____
_____
_____
_____

Related symptoms: _____

_____
_____
_____
_____
_____
_____

Secondary concern: _____

_____
_____
_____
_____
_____
_____

Related symptoms: _____

_____
_____
_____
_____
_____
_____

Follow-up from last appointment: _____

_____
_____
_____
_____
_____
_____

DURING/AFTER APPOINTMENT

DATE: _____

Doctor's advice on primary concern:_____

_____
_____
_____
_____
_____
_____

Doctor's advice on secondary concern:_____

_____
_____
_____
_____
_____
_____

Other notes:

_____
_____
_____
_____
_____
_____
_____
_____
_____
_____
_____
_____
_____
_____
_____
_____
_____
_____
_____
_____
_____
_____

BEFORE THE APPOINTMENT   APPOINTMENT DATE: _____

Name of Doctor: _____

Specialty: _____

Primary concern: _____
_____
_____
_____
_____
_____
_____

Related symptoms: _____
_____
_____
_____
_____
_____
_____

Secondary concern: _____
_____
_____
_____
_____
_____
_____

Related symptoms: _____
_____
_____
_____
_____
_____
_____

Follow-up from last appointment: _____
_____
_____
_____
_____
_____
_____

DURING/AFTER APPOINTMENT   DATE: _____

Doctor's advice on primary concern:_____

_____
_____
_____
_____
_____
_____

Doctor's advice on secondary concern:_____

_____
_____
_____
_____
_____
_____

Other notes:

_____
_____
_____
_____
_____
_____
_____
_____
_____
_____
_____
_____
_____
_____
_____
_____
_____
_____
_____
_____
_____
_____

BEFORE THE APPOINTMENT   APPOINTMENT DATE: _____

Name of Doctor: _____

Specialty: _____

Primary concern: _____
_____
_____
_____
_____
_____
_____

Related symptoms: _____
_____
_____
_____
_____
_____
_____

Secondary concern: _____
_____
_____
_____
_____
_____

Related symptoms: _____
_____
_____
_____
_____
_____

Follow-up from last appointment: _____
_____
_____
_____
_____
_____

DURING/AFTER APPOINTMENT

DATE: _____

Doctor's advice on primary concern:_____

_____
_____
_____
_____
_____
_____

Doctor's advice on secondary concern:_____

_____
_____
_____
_____
_____

Other notes:

_____
_____
_____
_____
_____
_____
_____
_____
_____
_____
_____
_____
_____
_____
_____
_____
_____
_____
_____
_____

BEFORE THE APPOINTMENT   APPOINTMENT DATE: _____

Name of Doctor: _____
Specialty: _____

Primary concern: _____
_____
_____
_____
_____
_____
_____

Related symptoms:_____
_____
_____
_____
_____
_____
_____

Secondary concern:_____
_____
_____
_____
_____
_____
_____

Related symptoms:_____
_____
_____
_____
_____
_____
_____

Follow-up from last appointment:_____
_____
_____
_____
_____
_____
_____

DURING/AFTER APPOINTMENT   DATE: _____

Doctor's advice on primary concern:_____

_____
_____
_____
_____
_____
_____

Doctor's advice on secondary concern:_____

_____
_____
_____
_____
_____
_____

Other notes:

_____
_____
_____
_____
_____
_____
_____
_____
_____
_____
_____
_____
_____
_____
_____
_____
_____
_____
_____
_____
_____

BEFORE THE APPOINTMENT   APPOINTMENT DATE: _____

Name of Doctor: _____

Specialty: _____

Primary concern: _____

_____
_____
_____
_____
_____
_____

Related symptoms: _____

_____
_____
_____
_____
_____
_____
_____

Secondary concern: _____

_____
_____
_____
_____
_____
_____

Related symptoms: _____

_____
_____
_____
_____
_____
_____

Follow-up from last appointment: _____

_____
_____
_____
_____
_____
_____

DURING/AFTER APPOINTMENT   DATE: _____

Doctor's advice on primary concern:_____
_____
_____
_____
_____
_____
_____

Doctor's advice on secondary concern:_____
_____
_____
_____
_____
_____
_____

Other notes:
_____
_____
_____
_____
_____
_____
_____
_____
_____
_____
_____
_____
_____
_____
_____
_____
_____
_____
_____
_____
_____
_____
_____
_____
_____

BEFORE THE APPOINTMENT   APPOINTMENT DATE: _____

Name of Doctor: _____
Specialty: _____

Primary concern: _____
_____
_____
_____
_____
_____
_____

Related symptoms:_____
_____
_____
_____
_____
_____
_____

Secondary concern:_____
_____
_____
_____
_____
_____

Related symptoms:_____
_____
_____
_____
_____
_____
_____

Follow-up from last appointment:_____
_____
_____
_____
_____
_____

DURING/AFTER APPOINTMENT   DATE: _____

Doctor's advice on primary concern:_____
_____
_____
_____
_____
_____
_____

Doctor's advice on secondary concern:_____
_____
_____
_____
_____
_____
_____

Other notes:
_____
_____
_____
_____
_____
_____
_____
_____
_____
_____
_____
_____
_____
_____
_____
_____
_____
_____
_____
_____
_____
_____
_____

FORE THE APPOINTMENT   APPOINTMENT DATE: _____

Name of Doctor: _____

Specialty: _____

Primary concern: _____
_____
_____
_____
_____
_____
_____

Related symptoms: _____
_____
_____
_____
_____
_____
_____

Secondary concern: _____
_____
_____
_____
_____
_____
_____

Related symptoms: _____
_____
_____
_____
_____
_____
_____

Follow-up from last appointment: _____
_____
_____
_____
_____
_____
_____

DURING/AFTER APPOINTMENT   DATE: _____

Doctor's advice on primary concern:_____

_____
_____
_____
_____
_____
_____

Doctor's advice on secondary concern:_____

_____
_____
_____
_____
_____
_____

Other notes:

_____
_____
_____
_____
_____
_____
_____
_____
_____
_____
_____
_____
_____
_____
_____
_____
_____
_____
_____
_____
_____
_____
_____

BEFORE THE APPOINTMENT   APPOINTMENT DATE: _____

Name of Doctor: _____
Specialty: _____

Primary concern: _____
_____
_____
_____
_____
_____
_____

Related symptoms: _____
_____
_____
_____
_____
_____
_____

Secondary concern: _____
_____
_____
_____
_____
_____
_____

Related symptoms: _____
_____
_____
_____
_____
_____
_____

Follow-up from last appointment: _____
_____
_____
_____
_____
_____

DURING/AFTER APPOINTMENT   DATE: _____

Doctor's advice on primary concern:_____

_____
_____
_____
_____
_____
_____

Doctor's advice on secondary concern:_____

_____
_____
_____
_____
_____
_____

Other notes:

_____
_____
_____
_____
_____
_____
_____
_____
_____
_____
_____
_____
_____
_____
_____
_____
_____
_____
_____
_____

BEFORE THE APPOINTMENT   APPOINTMENT DATE: _____

Name of Doctor: _____
Specialty: _____

Primary concern: _____
_____
_____
_____
_____
_____
_____

Related symptoms: _____
_____
_____
_____
_____
_____
_____

Secondary concern: _____
_____
_____
_____
_____
_____
_____

Related symptoms: _____
_____
_____
_____
_____
_____
_____

Follow-up from last appointment: _____
_____
_____
_____
_____
_____
_____

DURING/AFTER APPOINTMENT   DATE: _____

Doctor's advice on primary concern:_____

_____
_____
_____
_____
_____
_____

Doctor's advice on secondary concern:_____

_____
_____
_____
_____
_____
_____

Other notes:

_____
_____
_____
_____
_____
_____
_____
_____
_____
_____
_____
_____
_____
_____
_____
_____
_____
_____
_____
_____
_____
_____
_____

BEFORE THE APPOINTMENT   APPOINTMENT DATE: _____

Name of Doctor: _____
Specialty: _____

Primary concern: _____
_____
_____
_____
_____
_____
_____

Related symptoms: _____
_____
_____
_____
_____
_____
_____

Secondary concern: _____
_____
_____
_____
_____
_____
_____

Related symptoms: _____
_____
_____
_____
_____
_____
_____

Follow-up from last appointment: _____
_____
_____
_____
_____
_____

DURING/AFTER APPOINTMENT   DATE: _____

Doctor's advice on primary concern:_____

_____
_____
_____
_____
_____
_____

Doctor's advice on secondary concern:_____

_____
_____
_____
_____
_____
_____

Other notes:

_____
_____
_____
_____
_____
_____
_____
_____
_____
_____
_____
_____
_____
_____
_____
_____
_____
_____
_____
_____
_____
_____
_____

BEFORE THE APPOINTMENT   APPOINTMENT DATE: _____

Name of Doctor: _____
Specialty: _____

Primary concern: _____
_____
_____
_____
_____
_____
_____

Related symptoms:_____
_____
_____
_____
_____
_____
_____

Secondary concern:_____
_____
_____
_____
_____
_____
_____

Related symptoms:_____
_____
_____
_____
_____
_____
_____

Follow-up from last appointment:_____
_____
_____
_____
_____
_____
_____

DURING/AFTER APPOINTMENT

DATE: _____

Doctor's advice on primary concern:_____

_____
_____
_____
_____
_____
_____

Doctor's advice on secondary concern:_____

_____
_____
_____
_____
_____
_____

Other notes:

_____
_____
_____
_____
_____
_____
_____
_____
_____
_____
_____
_____
_____
_____
_____
_____
_____
_____
_____
_____
_____
_____

BEFORE THE APPOINTMENT   APPOINTMENT DATE: _____

Name of Doctor: _____
Specialty: _____

   Primary concern: _____
_____
_____
_____
_____
_____
_____

   Related symptoms:_____
_____
_____
_____
_____
_____
_____

   Secondary concern:_____
_____
_____
_____
_____
_____
_____

   Related symptoms:_____
_____
_____
_____
_____
_____
_____

   Follow-up from last appointment:_____
_____
_____
_____
_____
_____
_____

DURING/AFTER APPOINTMENT   DATE: _____

Doctor's advice on primary concern:_____
_____
_____
_____
_____
_____
_____

Doctor's advice on secondary concern:_____
_____
_____
_____
_____
_____
_____

Other notes:
_____
_____
_____
_____
_____
_____
_____
_____
_____
_____
_____
_____
_____
_____
_____
_____
_____
_____
_____
_____
_____
_____

BEFORE THE APPOINTMENT   APPOINTMENT DATE: _____

Name of Doctor: _____

Specialty: _____

Primary concern: _____

_____
_____
_____
_____
_____
_____

Related symptoms: _____

_____
_____
_____
_____
_____
_____

Secondary concern: _____

_____
_____
_____
_____
_____

Related symptoms: _____

_____
_____
_____
_____
_____
_____

Follow-up from last appointment: _____

_____
_____
_____
_____
_____

DURING/AFTER APPOINTMENT   DATE: _____

Doctor's advice on primary concern:_____
_____
_____
_____
_____
_____
_____

Doctor's advice on secondary concern:_____
_____
_____
_____
_____
_____
_____

Other notes:
_____
_____
_____
_____
_____
_____
_____
_____
_____
_____
_____
_____
_____
_____
_____
_____
_____
_____
_____
_____
_____
_____
_____

BEFORE THE APPOINTMENT   APPOINTMENT DATE: _____

Name of Doctor: _____

Specialty: _____

Primary concern: _____

_____
_____
_____
_____
_____
_____

Related symptoms:_____

_____
_____
_____
_____
_____
_____

Secondary concern:_____

_____
_____
_____
_____
_____
_____

Related symptoms:_____

_____
_____
_____
_____
_____
_____

Follow-up from last appointment:_____

_____
_____
_____
_____
_____

DURING/AFTER APPOINTMENT

DATE: _____

Doctor's advice on primary concern:_____

_____
_____
_____
_____
_____
_____

Doctor's advice on secondary concern:_____

_____
_____
_____
_____
_____
_____

Other notes:

_____
_____
_____
_____
_____
_____
_____
_____
_____
_____
_____
_____
_____
_____
_____
_____
_____
_____
_____
_____
_____
_____
_____

BEFORE THE APPOINTMENT   APPOINTMENT DATE: _____

Name of Doctor: _____

Specialty: _____

Primary concern: _____
_____
_____
_____
_____
_____
_____

Related symptoms:_____
_____
_____
_____
_____
_____
_____

Secondary concern:_____
_____
_____
_____
_____
_____
_____

Related symptoms:_____
_____
_____
_____
_____
_____
_____

Follow-up from last appointment:_____
_____
_____
_____
_____
_____

DURING/AFTER APPOINTMENT

DATE: _____

Doctor's advice on primary concern: _____
_____
_____
_____
_____
_____
_____
_____

Doctor's advice on secondary concern: _____
_____
_____
_____
_____
_____
_____

Other notes:
_____
_____
_____
_____
_____
_____
_____
_____
_____
_____
_____
_____
_____
_____
_____
_____
_____
_____
_____
_____
_____

BEFORE THE APPOINTMENT   APPOINTMENT DATE: _____

Name of Doctor: _____

Specialty: _____

Primary concern: _____

_____
_____
_____
_____
_____
_____

Related symptoms:_____

_____
_____
_____
_____
_____
_____

Secondary concern:_____

_____
_____
_____
_____
_____
_____

Related symptoms:_____

_____
_____
_____
_____
_____

Follow-up from last appointment:_____

_____
_____
_____
_____
_____

DURING/AFTER APPOINTMENT   DATE: _____

Doctor's advice on primary concern:_____

_____
_____
_____
_____
_____
_____

Doctor's advice on secondary concern:_____

_____
_____
_____
_____
_____
_____

Other notes:

_____
_____
_____
_____
_____
_____
_____
_____
_____
_____
_____
_____
_____
_____
_____
_____
_____
_____
_____
_____
_____
_____
_____
_____

BEFORE THE APPOINTMENT   APPOINTMENT DATE: _____

Name of Doctor: _____
Specialty: _____

Primary concern: _____
_____
_____
_____
_____
_____
_____

Related symptoms: _____
_____
_____
_____
_____
_____
_____

Secondary concern: _____
_____
_____
_____
_____
_____
_____

Related symptoms: _____
_____
_____
_____
_____
_____
_____

Follow-up from last appointment: _____
_____
_____
_____
_____
_____

DURING/AFTER APPOINTMENT   DATE: _____

Doctor's advice on primary concern:_____

_____
_____
_____
_____
_____
_____

Doctor's advice on secondary concern:_____

_____
_____
_____
_____
_____
_____

Other notes:

_____
_____
_____
_____
_____
_____
_____
_____
_____
_____
_____
_____
_____
_____
_____
_____
_____
_____
_____
_____
_____
_____
_____
_____
_____

BEFORE THE APPOINTMENT   APPOINTMENT DATE: _____

Name of Doctor: _____
Specialty: _____

Primary concern: _____
_____
_____
_____
_____
_____
_____

Related symptoms: _____
_____
_____
_____
_____
_____
_____

Secondary concern: _____
_____
_____
_____
_____
_____

Related symptoms: _____
_____
_____
_____
_____
_____

Follow-up from last appointment: _____
_____
_____
_____
_____
_____

DURING/AFTER APPOINTMENT   DATE: _____

Doctor's advice on primary concern:_____

_____
_____
_____
_____
_____
_____

Doctor's advice on secondary concern:_____

_____
_____
_____
_____
_____
_____

Other notes:

_____
_____
_____
_____
_____
_____
_____
_____
_____
_____
_____
_____
_____
_____
_____
_____
_____
_____
_____
_____
_____

BEFORE THE APPOINTMENT   APPOINTMENT DATE: _____

Name of Doctor: _____

Specialty: _____

Primary concern: _____

_____
_____
_____
_____
_____
_____

Related symptoms:_____

_____
_____
_____
_____
_____
_____

Secondary concern:_____

_____
_____
_____
_____
_____
_____

Related symptoms:_____

_____
_____
_____
_____
_____

Follow-up from last appointment:_____

_____
_____
_____
_____
_____

DURING/AFTER APPOINTMENT   DATE: _____

Doctor's advice on primary concern:_____

_____
_____
_____
_____
_____
_____
_____

Doctor's advice on secondary concern:_____

_____
_____
_____
_____
_____
_____
_____

Other notes:

_____
_____
_____
_____
_____
_____
_____
_____
_____
_____
_____
_____
_____
_____
_____
_____
_____
_____
_____
_____
_____
_____
_____
_____

BEFORE THE APPOINTMENT   APPOINTMENT DATE: _____

Name of Doctor: _____
Specialty: _____

Primary concern: _____
_____
_____
_____
_____
_____
_____

Related symptoms: _____
_____
_____
_____
_____
_____
_____

Secondary concern: _____
_____
_____
_____
_____
_____

Related symptoms: _____
_____
_____
_____
_____
_____

Follow-up from last appointment: _____
_____
_____
_____
_____
_____

DURING/AFTER APPOINTMENT   DATE: _____

Doctor's advice on primary concern:_____

_____
_____
_____
_____
_____
_____

Doctor's advice on secondary concern:_____

_____
_____
_____
_____
_____
_____

Other notes:

_____
_____
_____
_____
_____
_____
_____
_____
_____
_____
_____
_____
_____
_____
_____
_____
_____
_____
_____
_____
_____
_____

BEFORE THE APPOINTMENT   APPOINTMENT DATE: _____

Name of Doctor: _____
Specialty: _____

Primary concern: _____
_____
_____
_____
_____
_____
_____

Related symptoms: _____
_____
_____
_____
_____
_____
_____

Secondary concern: _____
_____
_____
_____
_____
_____

Related symptoms: _____
_____
_____
_____
_____
_____

Follow-up from last appointment: _____
_____
_____
_____
_____
_____

DURING/AFTER APPOINTMENT   DATE: _____

Doctor's advice on primary concern:_____

_____

_____

_____

_____

_____

_____

Doctor's advice on secondary concern:_____

_____

_____

_____

_____

_____

_____

Other notes:

_____

_____

_____

_____

_____

_____

_____

_____

_____

_____

_____

_____

_____

_____

_____

_____

_____

_____

_____

_____

_____

_____

BEFORE THE APPOINTMENT   APPOINTMENT DATE: _____

Name of Doctor: _____

Specialty: _____

Primary concern: _____
_____
_____
_____
_____
_____
_____

Related symptoms: _____
_____
_____
_____
_____
_____
_____

Secondary concern: _____
_____
_____
_____
_____
_____
_____

Related symptoms: _____
_____
_____
_____
_____
_____
_____

Follow-up from last appointment: _____
_____
_____
_____
_____
_____
_____

DURING/AFTER APPOINTMENT   DATE: _____

Doctor's advice on primary concern:_____
_____
_____
_____
_____
_____
_____

Doctor's advice on secondary concern:_____
_____
_____
_____
_____
_____
_____

Other notes:
_____
_____
_____
_____
_____
_____
_____
_____
_____
_____
_____
_____
_____
_____
_____
_____
_____
_____
_____
_____
_____
_____

BEFORE THE APPOINTMENT   APPOINTMENT DATE: _____

Name of Doctor: _____
Specialty: _____

Primary concern: _____
_____
_____
_____
_____
_____
_____

Related symptoms:_____
_____
_____
_____
_____
_____
_____

Secondary concern:_____
_____
_____
_____
_____
_____
_____

Related symptoms:_____
_____
_____
_____
_____
_____
_____

Follow-up from last appointment:_____
_____
_____
_____
_____
_____

DURING/AFTER APPOINTMENT

DATE: _____

Doctor's advice on primary concern: _____

_____

_____

_____

_____

_____

_____

Doctor's advice on secondary concern: _____

_____

_____

_____

_____

_____

Other notes:

_____

_____

_____

_____

_____

_____

_____

_____

_____

_____

_____

_____

_____

_____

_____

_____

_____

_____

BEFORE THE APPOINTMENT   APPOINTMENT DATE: _____

Name of Doctor: _____

Specialty: _____

Primary concern: _____

_____
_____
_____
_____
_____
_____

Related symptoms: _____

_____
_____
_____
_____
_____
_____
_____

Secondary concern: _____

_____
_____
_____
_____
_____
_____

Related symptoms: _____

_____
_____
_____
_____
_____
_____

Follow-up from last appointment: _____

_____
_____
_____
_____
_____
_____

DURING/AFTER APPOINTMENT   DATE: _____

Doctor's advice on primary concern:_____
_____
_____
_____
_____
_____
_____

Doctor's advice on secondary concern:_____
_____
_____
_____
_____
_____
_____

Other notes:
_____
_____
_____
_____
_____
_____
_____
_____
_____
_____
_____
_____
_____
_____
_____
_____
_____
_____
_____
_____
_____
_____

BEFORE THE APPOINTMENT   APPOINTMENT DATE: _____

Name of Doctor: _____

Specialty: _____

Primary concern: _____

_____
_____
_____
_____
_____
_____

Related symptoms:_____

_____
_____
_____
_____
_____
_____

Secondary concern:_____

_____
_____
_____
_____
_____
_____

Related symptoms:_____

_____
_____
_____
_____
_____
_____

Follow-up from last appointment:_____

_____
_____
_____
_____
_____
_____

DURING/AFTER APPOINTMENT   DATE: _____

Doctor's advice on primary concern:_____

_____
_____
_____
_____
_____
_____

Doctor's advice on secondary concern:_____

_____
_____
_____
_____
_____
_____

Other notes:

_____
_____
_____
_____
_____
_____
_____
_____
_____
_____
_____
_____
_____
_____
_____
_____
_____
_____
_____
_____
_____
_____
_____
_____

BEFORE THE APPOINTMENT   APPOINTMENT DATE: _____

Name of Doctor: _____

Specialty: _____

Primary concern: _____

_____
_____
_____
_____
_____
_____

Related symptoms: _____

_____
_____
_____
_____
_____
_____

Secondary concern: _____

_____
_____
_____
_____
_____
_____

Related symptoms: _____

_____
_____
_____
_____
_____
_____

Follow-up from last appointment: _____

_____
_____
_____
_____
_____
_____

DURING/AFTER APPOINTMENT   DATE: _____

Doctor's advice on primary concern:_____

_____
_____
_____
_____
_____
_____

Doctor's advice on secondary concern:_____

_____
_____
_____
_____
_____
_____

Other notes:

_____
_____
_____
_____
_____
_____
_____
_____
_____
_____
_____
_____
_____
_____
_____
_____
_____
_____
_____
_____
_____
_____

BEFORE THE APPOINTMENT   APPOINTMENT DATE: _____

Name of Doctor: _____
Specialty: _____

Primary concern: _____
_____
_____
_____
_____
_____
_____

Related symptoms: _____
_____
_____
_____
_____
_____
_____

Secondary concern: _____
_____
_____
_____
_____
_____
_____

Related symptoms: _____
_____
_____
_____
_____
_____
_____

Follow-up from last appointment: _____
_____
_____
_____
_____
_____
_____

DURING/AFTER APPOINTMENT   DATE: _____

Doctor's advice on primary concern:_____
_____
_____
_____
_____
_____
_____

Doctor's advice on secondary concern:_____
_____
_____
_____
_____
_____
_____

Other notes:
_____
_____
_____
_____
_____
_____
_____
_____
_____
_____
_____
_____
_____
_____
_____
_____
_____
_____
_____
_____
_____
_____

BEFORE THE APPOINTMENT   APPOINTMENT DATE: _____

Name of Doctor: _____

Specialty: _____

Primary concern: _____
_____
_____
_____
_____
_____
_____

Related symptoms:_____
_____
_____
_____
_____
_____
_____

Secondary concern:_____
_____
_____
_____
_____
_____

Related symptoms:_____
_____
_____
_____
_____
_____

Follow-up from last appointment:_____
_____
_____
_____
_____
_____

DURING/AFTER APPOINTMENT   DATE: _____

Doctor's advice on primary concern:_____
_____
_____
_____
_____
_____
_____

Doctor's advice on secondary concern:_____
_____
_____
_____
_____
_____
_____

Other notes:
_____
_____
_____
_____
_____
_____
_____
_____
_____
_____
_____
_____
_____
_____
_____
_____
_____
_____
_____
_____
_____
_____

BEFORE THE APPOINTMENT   APPOINTMENT DATE: _____

Name of Doctor: _____

Specialty: _____

   Primary concern: _____

_____
_____
_____
_____
_____
_____

   Related symptoms:_____

_____
_____
_____
_____
_____
_____

   Secondary concern:_____

_____
_____
_____
_____
_____
_____

   Related symptoms:_____

_____
_____
_____
_____
_____

   Follow-up from last appointment:_____

_____
_____
_____
_____
_____

DURING/AFTER APPOINTMENT   DATE: _____

Doctor's advice on primary concern:_____

_____

_____

_____

_____

_____

_____

Doctor's advice on secondary concern:_____

_____

_____

_____

_____

_____

_____

Other notes:

_____

_____

_____

_____

_____

_____

_____

_____

_____

_____

_____

_____

_____

_____

_____

_____

_____

_____

_____

_____

_____

_____

BEFORE THE APPOINTMENT   APPOINTMENT DATE: _____

Name of Doctor: _____

Specialty: _____

Primary concern: _____

_____
_____
_____
_____
_____
_____

Related symptoms:_____

_____
_____
_____
_____
_____
_____

Secondary concern:_____

_____
_____
_____
_____
_____
_____

Related symptoms:_____

_____
_____
_____
_____
_____
_____

Follow-up from last appointment:_____

_____
_____
_____
_____
_____

DURING/AFTER APPOINTMENT

DATE: _____

Doctor's advice on primary concern:_____
_____
_____
_____
_____
_____
_____

Doctor's advice on secondary concern:_____
_____
_____
_____
_____
_____

Other notes:
_____
_____
_____
_____
_____
_____
_____
_____
_____
_____
_____
_____
_____
_____
_____
_____
_____
_____
_____
_____
_____
_____
_____

BEFORE THE APPOINTMENT   APPOINTMENT DATE: _____

Name of Doctor: _____

Specialty: _____

Primary concern: _____

_____

_____

_____

_____

_____

_____

Related symptoms: _____

_____

_____

_____

_____

_____

_____

Secondary concern: _____

_____

_____

_____

_____

_____

_____

Related symptoms: _____

_____

_____

_____

_____

_____

_____

Follow-up from last appointment: _____

_____

_____

_____

_____

_____

DURING/AFTER APPOINTMENT

DATE: _____

Doctor's advice on primary concern: _____
_____
_____
_____
_____
_____
_____

Doctor's advice on secondary concern: _____
_____
_____
_____
_____
_____
_____

Other notes:
_____
_____
_____
_____
_____
_____
_____
_____
_____
_____
_____
_____
_____
_____
_____
_____
_____
_____
_____
_____
_____
_____
_____
_____
_____

BEFORE THE APPOINTMENT   APPOINTMENT DATE: _____

Name of Doctor: _____

Specialty: _____

Primary concern: _____

_____
_____
_____
_____
_____
_____

Related symptoms: _____

_____
_____
_____
_____
_____
_____

Secondary concern: _____

_____
_____
_____
_____
_____
_____

Related symptoms: _____

_____
_____
_____
_____
_____
_____

Follow-up from last appointment: _____

_____
_____
_____
_____
_____
_____

DURING/AFTER APPOINTMENT   DATE: _____

Doctor's advice on primary concern:_____

_____
_____
_____
_____
_____
_____

Doctor's advice on secondary concern:_____

_____
_____
_____
_____
_____
_____

Other notes:

_____
_____
_____
_____
_____
_____
_____
_____
_____
_____
_____
_____
_____
_____
_____
_____
_____
_____
_____
_____
_____
_____
_____

BEFORE THE APPOINTMENT   APPOINTMENT DATE: _____

Name of Doctor: _____

Specialty: _____

Primary concern: _____

_____

_____

_____

_____

_____

_____

Related symptoms: _____

_____

_____

_____

_____

_____

_____

Secondary concern: _____

_____

_____

_____

_____

_____

_____

Related symptoms: _____

_____

_____

_____

_____

_____

_____

Follow-up from last appointment: _____

_____

_____

_____

_____

_____

_____

DURING/AFTER APPOINTMENT

DATE: _____

Doctor's advice on primary concern:_____
_____
_____
_____
_____
_____
_____

Doctor's advice on secondary concern:_____
_____
_____
_____
_____
_____
_____

Other notes:
_____
_____
_____
_____
_____
_____
_____
_____
_____
_____
_____
_____
_____
_____
_____
_____
_____
_____
_____
_____
_____
_____

BEFORE THE APPOINTMENT   APPOINTMENT DATE: _____

Name of Doctor: _____

Specialty: _____

Primary concern: _____
_____
_____
_____
_____
_____
_____

Related symptoms:_____
_____
_____
_____
_____
_____
_____

Secondary concern:_____
_____
_____
_____
_____
_____

Related symptoms:_____
_____
_____
_____
_____
_____

Follow-up from last appointment:_____
_____
_____
_____
_____
_____

DURING/AFTER APPOINTMENT   DATE: _____

Doctor's advice on primary concern:_____

_____
_____
_____
_____
_____
_____

Doctor's advice on secondary concern:_____

_____
_____
_____
_____
_____
_____

Other notes:

_____
_____
_____
_____
_____
_____
_____
_____
_____
_____
_____
_____
_____
_____
_____
_____
_____
_____
_____
_____
_____

BEFORE THE APPOINTMENT   APPOINTMENT DATE: _____

Name of Doctor: _____
Specialty: _____

Primary concern: _____
_____
_____
_____
_____
_____
_____

Related symptoms: _____
_____
_____
_____
_____
_____
_____

Secondary concern: _____
_____
_____
_____
_____
_____
_____

Related symptoms: _____
_____
_____
_____
_____
_____
_____

Follow-up from last appointment: _____
_____
_____
_____
_____
_____
_____

DURING/AFTER APPOINTMENT   DATE: _____

Doctor's advice on primary concern:_____

_____
_____
_____
_____
_____
_____

Doctor's advice on secondary concern:_____

_____
_____
_____
_____
_____
_____

Other notes:

_____
_____
_____
_____
_____
_____
_____
_____
_____
_____
_____
_____
_____
_____
_____
_____
_____
_____
_____
_____
_____
_____
_____

BEFORE THE APPOINTMENT   APPOINTMENT DATE: _____

Name of Doctor: _____
Specialty: _____

Primary concern: _____
_____
_____
_____
_____
_____
_____

Related symptoms:_____
_____
_____
_____
_____
_____
_____

Secondary concern:_____
_____
_____
_____
_____
_____
_____

Related symptoms:_____
_____
_____
_____
_____
_____
_____

Follow-up from last appointment:_____
_____
_____
_____
_____
_____
_____

DURING/AFTER APPOINTMENT   DATE: _____

Doctor's advice on primary concern:_____

_____
_____
_____
_____
_____
_____

Doctor's advice on secondary concern:_____

_____
_____
_____
_____
_____
_____

Other notes:

_____
_____
_____
_____
_____
_____
_____
_____
_____
_____
_____
_____
_____
_____
_____
_____
_____
_____
_____
_____

BEFORE THE APPOINTMENT   APPOINTMENT DATE: _____

Name of Doctor: _____

Specialty: _____

Primary concern: _____

_____
_____
_____
_____
_____
_____

Related symptoms: _____

_____
_____
_____
_____
_____
_____

Secondary concern: _____

_____
_____
_____
_____
_____
_____

Related symptoms: _____

_____
_____
_____
_____
_____
_____

Follow-up from last appointment: _____

_____
_____
_____
_____
_____

DURING/AFTER APPOINTMENT   DATE: _____

Doctor's advice on primary concern:_____
_____
_____
_____
_____
_____
_____

Doctor's advice on secondary concern:_____
_____
_____
_____
_____
_____
_____

Other notes:
_____
_____
_____
_____
_____
_____
_____
_____
_____
_____
_____
_____
_____
_____
_____
_____
_____
_____
_____
_____
_____

BEFORE THE APPOINTMENT   APPOINTMENT DATE: _____

Name of Doctor: _____
Specialty: _____

Primary concern: _____
_____
_____
_____
_____
_____
_____

Related symptoms:_____
_____
_____
_____
_____
_____
_____

Secondary concern:_____
_____
_____
_____
_____
_____
_____

Related symptoms:_____
_____
_____
_____
_____
_____
_____

Follow-up from last appointment:_____
_____
_____
_____
_____
_____
_____

DURING/AFTER APPOINTMENT   DATE: _____

Doctor's advice on primary concern:_____
_____
_____
_____
_____
_____
_____

Doctor's advice on secondary concern:_____
_____
_____
_____
_____
_____
_____

Other notes:
_____
_____
_____
_____
_____
_____
_____
_____
_____
_____
_____
_____
_____
_____
_____
_____
_____
_____
_____
_____

BEFORE THE APPOINTMENT   APPOINTMENT DATE: _____

Name of Doctor: _____

Specialty: _____

Primary concern: _____
_____
_____
_____
_____
_____
_____

Related symptoms: _____
_____
_____
_____
_____
_____
_____

Secondary concern: _____
_____
_____
_____
_____
_____
_____

Related symptoms: _____
_____
_____
_____
_____
_____

Follow-up from last appointment: _____
_____
_____
_____
_____
_____

DURING/AFTER APPOINTMENT   DATE: _____

Doctor's advice on primary concern:_____
_____
_____
_____
_____
_____
_____
_____

Doctor's advice on secondary concern:_____
_____
_____
_____
_____
_____
_____

Other notes:
_____
_____
_____
_____
_____
_____
_____
_____
_____
_____
_____
_____
_____
_____
_____
_____
_____
_____
_____
_____

BEFORE THE APPOINTMENT   APPOINTMENT DATE: _____

Name of Doctor: _____

Specialty: _____

Primary concern: _____
_____
_____
_____
_____
_____
_____

Related symptoms: _____
_____
_____
_____
_____
_____
_____

Secondary concern: _____
_____
_____
_____
_____
_____

Related symptoms: _____
_____
_____
_____
_____
_____

Follow-up from last appointment: _____
_____
_____
_____
_____
_____

DURING/AFTER APPOINTMENT   DATE: _____

Doctor's advice on primary concern:_____

_____
_____
_____
_____
_____
_____

Doctor's advice on secondary concern:_____

_____
_____
_____
_____
_____
_____

Other notes:

_____
_____
_____
_____
_____
_____
_____
_____
_____
_____
_____
_____
_____
_____
_____
_____
_____
_____
_____
_____
_____
_____
_____
_____

BEFORE THE APPOINTMENT   APPOINTMENT DATE: _____

Name of Doctor: _____
Specialty: _____

Primary concern: _____
_____
_____
_____
_____
_____
_____

Related symptoms:_____
_____
_____
_____
_____
_____
_____

Secondary concern:_____
_____
_____
_____
_____
_____
_____

Related symptoms:_____
_____
_____
_____
_____
_____
_____

Follow-up from last appointment:_____
_____
_____
_____
_____
_____

DURING/AFTER APPOINTMENT   DATE: _____

Doctor's advice on primary concern:_____
_____
_____
_____
_____
_____
_____

Doctor's advice on secondary concern:_____
_____
_____
_____
_____
_____
_____

Other notes:
_____
_____
_____
_____
_____
_____
_____
_____
_____
_____
_____
_____
_____
_____
_____
_____
_____
_____
_____
_____
_____
_____

BEFORE THE APPOINTMENT   APPOINTMENT DATE: _____

Name of Doctor: _____
Specialty: _____

Primary concern: _____
_____
_____
_____
_____
_____
_____

Related symptoms:_____
_____
_____
_____
_____
_____
_____

Secondary concern:_____
_____
_____
_____
_____
_____
_____

Related symptoms:_____
_____
_____
_____
_____
_____

Follow-up from last appointment:_____
_____
_____
_____
_____
_____
_____

DURING/AFTER APPOINTMENT　　　DATE: _____

Doctor's advice on primary concern:_____
_____
_____
_____
_____
_____
_____

Doctor's advice on secondary concern:_____
_____
_____
_____
_____
_____
_____

Other notes:
_____
_____
_____
_____
_____
_____
_____
_____
_____
_____
_____
_____
_____
_____
_____
_____
_____
_____
_____
_____
_____
_____
_____

BEFORE THE APPOINTMENT   APPOINTMENT DATE: _____

Name of Doctor: _____

Specialty: _____

Primary concern: _____

_____

_____

_____

_____

_____

_____

Related symptoms: _____

_____

_____

_____

_____

_____

_____

Secondary concern: _____

_____

_____

_____

_____

_____

_____

Related symptoms: _____

_____

_____

_____

_____

_____

_____

Follow-up from last appointment: _____

_____

_____

_____

_____

_____

DURING/AFTER APPOINTMENT   DATE: _____

Doctor's advice on primary concern:_____
_____
_____
_____
_____
_____
_____

Doctor's advice on secondary concern:_____
_____
_____
_____
_____
_____
_____

Other notes:
_____
_____
_____
_____
_____
_____
_____
_____
_____
_____
_____
_____
_____
_____
_____
_____
_____
_____
_____
_____
_____
_____

BEFORE THE APPOINTMENT   APPOINTMENT DATE: _____

Name of Doctor: _____

Specialty: _____

Primary concern: _____
_____
_____
_____
_____
_____
_____

Related symptoms: _____
_____
_____
_____
_____
_____
_____

Secondary concern: _____
_____
_____
_____
_____
_____
_____

Related symptoms: _____
_____
_____
_____
_____
_____
_____

Follow-up from last appointment: _____
_____
_____
_____
_____
_____

DURING/AFTER APPOINTMENT   DATE: _____

Doctor's advice on primary concern:_____

_____
_____
_____
_____
_____
_____

Doctor's advice on secondary concern:_____

_____
_____
_____
_____
_____
_____

Other notes:

_____
_____
_____
_____
_____
_____
_____
_____
_____
_____
_____
_____
_____
_____
_____
_____
_____
_____
_____
_____
_____
_____
_____

BEFORE THE APPOINTMENT   APPOINTMENT DATE: _____

Name of Doctor: _____
Specialty: _____

Primary concern: _____
_____
_____
_____
_____
_____
_____

Related symptoms:_____
_____
_____
_____
_____
_____
_____

Secondary concern:_____
_____
_____
_____
_____
_____

Related symptoms:_____
_____
_____
_____
_____
_____

Follow-up from last appointment:_____
_____
_____
_____
_____
_____

DURING/AFTER APPOINTMENT

DATE: _____

Doctor's advice on primary concern:_____

_____
_____
_____
_____
_____
_____

Doctor's advice on secondary concern:_____

_____
_____
_____
_____
_____
_____

Other notes:

_____
_____
_____
_____
_____
_____
_____
_____
_____
_____
_____
_____
_____
_____
_____
_____
_____
_____
_____
_____
_____
_____
_____

BEFORE THE APPOINTMENT   APPOINTMENT DATE: _____

Name of Doctor: _____

Specialty: _____

Primary concern: _____

_____
_____
_____
_____
_____
_____

Related symptoms: _____

_____
_____
_____
_____
_____
_____

Secondary concern: _____

_____
_____
_____
_____
_____
_____

Related symptoms: _____

_____
_____
_____
_____
_____
_____

Follow-up from last appointment: _____

_____
_____
_____
_____
_____
_____

DURING/AFTER APPOINTMENT   DATE: _____

Doctor's advice on primary concern:_____
_____
_____
_____
_____
_____
_____

Doctor's advice on secondary concern:_____
_____
_____
_____
_____
_____
_____

Other notes:
_____
_____
_____
_____
_____
_____
_____
_____
_____
_____
_____
_____
_____
_____
_____
_____
_____
_____
_____
_____
_____
_____
_____
_____

BEFORE THE APPOINTMENT   APPOINTMENT DATE: _____

Name of Doctor: _____

Specialty: _____

Primary concern: _____

_____
_____
_____
_____
_____
_____

Related symptoms: _____

_____
_____
_____
_____
_____
_____

Secondary concern: _____

_____
_____
_____
_____
_____
_____

Related symptoms: _____

_____
_____
_____
_____
_____
_____

Follow-up from last appointment: _____

_____
_____
_____
_____
_____
_____

DURING/AFTER APPOINTMENT   DATE: _____

Doctor's advice on primary concern:_____

_____
_____
_____
_____
_____
_____

Doctor's advice on secondary concern:_____

_____
_____
_____
_____
_____
_____

Other notes:

_____
_____
_____
_____
_____
_____
_____
_____
_____
_____
_____
_____
_____
_____
_____
_____
_____
_____
_____
_____
_____
_____
_____

BEFORE THE APPOINTMENT   APPOINTMENT DATE: _____

Name of Doctor: _____

Specialty: _____

Primary concern: _____
_____
_____
_____
_____
_____
_____

Related symptoms: _____
_____
_____
_____
_____
_____
_____

Secondary concern: _____
_____
_____
_____
_____
_____
_____

Related symptoms: _____
_____
_____
_____
_____
_____
_____

Follow-up from last appointment: _____
_____
_____
_____
_____
_____
_____

DURING/AFTER APPOINTMENT   DATE: _____

Doctor's advice on primary concern:_____
_____
_____
_____
_____
_____
_____

Doctor's advice on secondary concern:_____
_____
_____
_____
_____
_____
_____

Other notes:
_____
_____
_____
_____
_____
_____
_____
_____
_____
_____
_____
_____
_____
_____
_____
_____
_____
_____
_____
_____
_____

BEFORE THE APPOINTMENT   APPOINTMENT DATE: _____

Name of Doctor: _____
Specialty: _____

Primary concern: _____
_____
_____
_____
_____
_____
_____

Related symptoms:_____
_____
_____
_____
_____
_____
_____

Secondary concern:_____
_____
_____
_____
_____
_____
_____

Related symptoms:_____
_____
_____
_____
_____
_____
_____

Follow-up from last appointment:_____
_____
_____
_____
_____
_____
_____

DURING/AFTER APPOINTMENT

DATE: _____

Doctor's advice on primary concern:_____

_____

_____

_____

_____

_____

_____

Doctor's advice on secondary concern:_____

_____

_____

_____

_____

_____

_____

Other notes:

_____

_____

_____

_____

_____

_____

_____

_____

_____

_____

_____

_____

_____

_____

_____

_____

_____

_____

_____

_____

_____

_____

_____

BEFORE THE APPOINTMENT   APPOINTMENT DATE: _____

Name of Doctor: _____

Specialty: _____

Primary concern: _____
_____
_____
_____
_____
_____
_____

Related symptoms: _____
_____
_____
_____
_____
_____
_____

Secondary concern: _____
_____
_____
_____
_____
_____

Related symptoms: _____
_____
_____
_____
_____
_____

Follow-up from last appointment: _____
_____
_____
_____
_____
_____

DURING/AFTER APPOINTMENT   DATE: _____

Doctor's advice on primary concern:_____
_____
_____
_____
_____
_____
_____

Doctor's advice on secondary concern:_____
_____
_____
_____
_____
_____
_____

Other notes:
_____
_____
_____
_____
_____
_____
_____
_____
_____
_____
_____
_____
_____
_____
_____
_____
_____
_____
_____
_____
_____
_____

BEFORE THE APPOINTMENT   APPOINTMENT DATE: _____

Name of Doctor: _____
Specialty: _____

Primary concern: _____
_____
_____
_____
_____
_____
_____

Related symptoms: _____
_____
_____
_____
_____
_____
_____

Secondary concern: _____
_____
_____
_____
_____
_____
_____

Related symptoms: _____
_____
_____
_____
_____
_____

Follow-up from last appointment: _____
_____
_____
_____
_____
_____
_____

DURING/AFTER APPOINTMENT

DATE: _____

Doctor's advice on primary concern: _____

_____

_____

_____

_____

_____

_____

Doctor's advice on secondary concern: _____

_____

_____

_____

_____

_____

_____

Other notes:

_____

_____

_____

_____

_____

_____

_____

_____

_____

_____

_____

_____

_____

_____

_____

_____

_____

_____

_____

_____

BEFORE THE APPOINTMENT   APPOINTMENT DATE: _____

Name of Doctor: _____
Specialty: _____

Primary concern: _____
_____
_____
_____
_____
_____
_____

Related symptoms:_____
_____
_____
_____
_____
_____
_____

Secondary concern:_____
_____
_____
_____
_____
_____

Related symptoms:_____
_____
_____
_____
_____
_____
_____

Follow-up from last appointment:_____
_____
_____
_____
_____
_____

DURING/AFTER APPOINTMENT   DATE: _____

Doctor's advice on primary concern:_____
_____
_____
_____
_____
_____
_____

Doctor's advice on secondary concern:_____
_____
_____
_____
_____
_____
_____

Other notes:
_____
_____
_____
_____
_____
_____
_____
_____
_____
_____
_____
_____
_____
_____
_____
_____
_____
_____
_____
_____
_____
_____
_____
_____

BEFORE THE APPOINTMENT   APPOINTMENT DATE: _____

Name of Doctor: _____

Specialty: _____

Primary concern: _____

_____
_____
_____
_____
_____
_____

Related symptoms: _____

_____
_____
_____
_____
_____
_____

Secondary concern: _____

_____
_____
_____
_____
_____
_____

Related symptoms: _____

_____
_____
_____
_____
_____
_____

Follow-up from last appointment: _____

_____
_____
_____
_____
_____
_____

DURING/AFTER APPOINTMENT   DATE: _____

Doctor's advice on primary concern: _____

_____
_____
_____
_____
_____
_____
_____

Doctor's advice on secondary concern: _____

_____
_____
_____
_____
_____
_____

Other notes:

_____
_____
_____
_____
_____
_____
_____
_____
_____
_____
_____
_____
_____
_____
_____
_____
_____
_____
_____
_____
_____
_____

BEFORE THE APPOINTMENT   APPOINTMENT DATE: _____

Name of Doctor: _____

Specialty: _____

Primary concern: _____

_____
_____
_____
_____
_____
_____

Related symptoms: _____

_____
_____
_____
_____
_____
_____

Secondary concern: _____

_____
_____
_____
_____
_____
_____

Related symptoms: _____

_____
_____
_____
_____
_____
_____

Follow-up from last appointment: _____

_____
_____
_____
_____
_____
_____

DURING/AFTER APPOINTMENT   DATE: _____

Doctor's advice on primary concern:_____

_____
_____
_____
_____
_____
_____

Doctor's advice on secondary concern:_____

_____
_____
_____
_____
_____
_____

Other notes:

_____
_____
_____
_____
_____
_____
_____
_____
_____
_____
_____
_____
_____
_____
_____
_____
_____
_____
_____
_____
_____
_____
_____

BEFORE THE APPOINTMENT   APPOINTMENT DATE: _____

Name of Doctor: _____

Specialty: _____

Primary concern: _____

_____
_____
_____
_____
_____
_____

Related symptoms: _____

_____
_____
_____
_____
_____
_____
_____

Secondary concern: _____

_____
_____
_____
_____
_____
_____

Related symptoms: _____

_____
_____
_____
_____
_____
_____

Follow-up from last appointment: _____

_____
_____
_____
_____
_____
_____

DURING/AFTER APPOINTMENT   DATE: _____

Doctor's advice on primary concern:_____
_____
_____
_____
_____
_____
_____
_____

Doctor's advice on secondary concern:_____
_____
_____
_____
_____
_____
_____

Other notes:
_____
_____
_____
_____
_____
_____
_____
_____
_____
_____
_____
_____
_____
_____
_____
_____
_____
_____
_____
_____
_____
_____
_____

BEFORE THE APPOINTMENT   APPOINTMENT DATE: _____

Name of Doctor: _____

Specialty: _____

Primary concern: _____
_____
_____
_____
_____
_____
_____

Related symptoms: _____
_____
_____
_____
_____
_____
_____

Secondary concern: _____
_____
_____
_____
_____
_____
_____

Related symptoms: _____
_____
_____
_____
_____
_____
_____

Follow-up from last appointment: _____
_____
_____
_____
_____
_____
_____

DURING/AFTER APPOINTMENT   DATE: _____

Doctor's advice on primary concern:_____
_____
_____
_____
_____
_____
_____

Doctor's advice on secondary concern:_____
_____
_____
_____
_____
_____
_____

Other notes:
_____
_____
_____
_____
_____
_____
_____
_____
_____
_____
_____
_____
_____
_____
_____
_____
_____
_____
_____
_____
_____
_____
_____

ABOUT THE CREATOR

Kaden Stillwell is a chronically ill millennial living in Portland, Oregon. They enjoy textile crafting (such as sewing, crochet, and weaving), activism, and video games (their favorites are Minecraft, Stardew Valley, and the Harvest Moon series). They made this book to help other chronically ill people keep track of the advice that comes from multiple doctors.

You can find more of their work, including coloring books, by searching "Kaden Stillwell" on Amazon.

Or, for non-book products, visit their wordpress site at kadencreates.wordpress.com

www.ingramcontent.com/pod-product-compliance
Lightning Source LLC
Chambersburg PA
CBHW081347280526
45788CB00009B/2798